Cycled Serenity

Mindful Road Cycling and Mountain Biking

Table of Contents

Chapter 1. Introduction

Dive into the rhythmic world of mindful cycling with our Special Report: 'Cycled Serenity: Mindful Road Cycling and Mountain Biking'. This engaging, refreshing grind into the nexus of physical activity and mindful consciousness will help you connect the dots between physical exhilaration and spiritual tranquility. Find serenity amidst the tumultuous chaos of your daily life by combining the restorative power of mindfulness with the thrill of road cycling and mountain biking. Whether you're a seasoned cyclist or a budding enthusiast, embark on a journey that promises to transform your regular rides into holistic experiences, packed with insights for your body, your mind, and your soul. Your adventure into a new perspective of wellbeing starts here. Prepare for a ride, unlike any other, that will make you look forward to every upcoming bend and hill, not just for the exhilarating rush but also for the peace that follows. Don't just cycle, learn to flow with your ride!

Chapter 2. The Intersection of Cycling and Mindfulness

Cycling is more than just a form of exercise; it is a therapeutic activity that simultaneously strengthens the body and calities the mind. Over the years, cycling has become synonymous with a sense of liberation, a retreat from the frenetic pace of our everyday lives. With each push of the pedal, every swoop down a rolling hill or meandering path, becomes an immersion into the present moment creating a seamless bridge between cycling and mindfulness.

2.1. The Power of Now through the Wheels

Right before the start, standing with your hand wrapped around the handlebar, the bike beneath you, you can already begin to engage with the present. As you shove off, feel the weight shift from your feet to the bike. Be mindful of that transition. As you begin to pedal, notice the chain's response, the connection between your body's action and the mechanical reaction past beneath the bike. This intermingling of energy and action is the initiation of your mindfulness journey.

The mindfulness begins to deepen as your ride progresses. Every pedal stroke calls you to the present moment. Feel your leg muscles contracting and releasing with each stroke, your feet steadily turning the pedals, your hands lightly gripping the handlebars. Your ride becomes a meditation in motion, a physical manifestation of living in the 'now.'

2.2. The Cadence of Breath and Pedals

Your breath and your pedal strokes naturally sync. As exertion increases, your breath accelerates, matching the rhythm of your pedaling. This synchronization creates a pulsating rhythm that can deepen your mindfulness experience. Become aware of your breath, the way your chest rises and falls, the rush of air in and out of your lungs. Each exhale can be a reminder to release tension; each inhale, an opportunity to draw in calm energy.

2.3. Cycling as a Sensorial Overload

Cycling allows you to absorb your surroundings through your senses. The wind rushes past your ears, the sun's rays touch your skin, the scenery unfolds around you. Let these sensory experiences draw you into the present moment. Notice the smells, the play of light and shadow, the temperature fluctuations as you pass under the shade of a tree or face the sun again.

2.4. Guiding Your Thoughts

Cycling is a rhythmic, repetitive activity - a fertile ground for mind wandering. But it's during these wandering moments where you can gently guide your thoughts back to the experience of cycling itself. Notice your form, your pedaling efficiency, or the bike's response to your input. Use each moment of awareness as an opportunity to dive deeper into the present, to connect with the essence of the ride.

2.5. Embracing the Challenges

Every uphill climb and rough pathway is a challenge calling for your mental strength. Here, mindfulness allows you to shift focus from the hardship towards the lessons and experiences these challenges bring. Embrace the sweat, the fatigue, the burn of a strenuous climb. Ponder on your dedication, your ability to engage with discomfort, and your continuous strive to become stronger. The satisfaction of overcoming these challenges brings about a sense of tranquility and accomplishment, strengthening your mental fortitude.

2.6. Cycling and Compassion

Alone or in a group, cycling fosters a sense of compassion and camaraderie. Every shared "hello" or nod with a fellow cyclist on the road can become a moment of mindful interaction. The shared experiences on the trail, be it hardships, or the simple joy of riding, foster deeper connections.

Connecting physical exhilaration with mindful consciousness, cycling becomes a catalyst for a deeper sense of well-being. It becomes more than just a rides—it becomes a means to physically engage with our surroundings, maintain our health, exercise our minds, deepen our awareness, and foster connections with ourselves and others. As the wheels continue to spin, so does our journey into serenity through cycling and mindfulness. In this rhythm, we find solace, peace, and a heightened awareness of life's pulsating energy.

Chapter 3. Road Cycling: Exploring Focus and Flow

First, let us venture into an understanding of road cycling's unique aspects and how it fosters a state of focus and flow.

3.1. The Unique Language of Road Cycling

Road cycling is more than just a means of transport or a way to burn calories. Its true essence lies in the rhythmic pattern of your legs pushing on the pedals, the humming sound of wheels on asphalt, and your focused interaction with the environment. Everything begins to blur out except the road ahead, your breath, and your beating heart. As the journey unfolds, your body learns a new language - a language that speaks through endurance, rhythm, balance, and intuition.

It is this language, a physical and mental dialogue, which helps in cultivating focus and flow, and transcending us into a state of mindfulness.

3.2. Understanding Focus and Flow in Cycling

When we consider the two key elements that make the mindful cycling experience - focus and flow - their relationship becomes fascinating. Focus is the ability to direct your attention toward the task at hand, in this case, cycling. Flow, on the other hand, is a state where you are fully immersed and involved in your cycling, rendering a sense of aligned energy and gratification.

Both these aspects interact and reinforce each other in the act of cycling. A heightened focus leads to better flow, while being in a state of flow increases one's level of focus. Together, they orchestrate a symphony in your mind that amplifies your senses, making the cycling experience consciously enriching.

3.3. Integrating Mindfulness into Road Cycling

As straightforward as the act of cycling may seem, integrating mindfulness into the process requires practice. The trick is to convert each pedal stroke into a mindful movement. You focus on the flow of your breath, the rhythm of your heart, the turning of your wheels, your grip on the handlebars, and the changing scenery. Each of these elements functions as an anchor, consistently bringing your attention back when it tends to wander.

Gradually, you begin to respond rather than react to what comes your way on the ride. An impeding hill is no longer an obstacle; instead, it turns into an opportunity to strengthen your resolve. A headwind is not a hindrance, but a prospect to test your endurance. This transformation from a reactive to a responsive state is what mindfulness in road cycling aspires to achieve.

3.4. Cycling and Breath: Synchronizing for Optimal Performance

The breath is often considered the bridge between the mind and the body. In road cycling, the breath becomes your most trusted ally. Syncing your breath with your cycling rhythm helps you achieve a smooth, controlled pace. As your breath deepens and becomes rhythmic, each exhalation drawing out more than just air but letting go of any tension in the body, a synergy between your inner and outer worlds takes place. This harmony lays the foundation for a flow state.

3.5. Mindful Strategies to Enhance your Road Cycling Experience

In gaining focus and flow, incorporating mindful strategies into your road cycling routine proves beneficial. These may vary from visualization techniques before your ride to simple actions like cleaning your bike mindfully, focusing on the intricate parts, and acknowledging its importance in your journey.

While on the ride, take intermittent breaks to be still, catching onto the subtle sounds and smells of the surroundings, and savoring these moments of tranquility.

3.6. Learning from the Ride: Transferring Mindfulness to Everyday Life

Mindful road cycling is not merely a practice confined to the duration of your ride. It extends beyond that, transforming the way we perceive our everyday life. The focus one develops and the flow one experiences become instrumental in mindfulness-based stress reduction (MBSR).

The habits formed during the mindful cycle rides overflow into routines. Be it waiting at a traffic signal, washing dishes, or attending a meeting, moments start turning into opportunities for being present.

In conclusion, road cycling serves as more than a physical activity. Its rhythmic, continuous nature combined with the discipline of focus and transcendence through flow provide everything one needs to enter a meditative state. Engaging in mindful road cycling is a journey towards self-awareness and resilience, transforming not only your cycling but navigating the contours of your personal and professional life with newfound clarity and peace. It's an invitation to not just cycle, but to truly become one with the ride.

Chapter 4. Mountain Biking: The Thrill of Mindful Challenges

The moments of anticipation just before the ride, the tightening of the helmet straps, the stretching of the fingers around the handlebar grips, the first press of the foot on the pedal; it's these sensations that grant mountain biking its status as an unparalleled journey enticing thrill-seekers and mindfulness practitioners alike. This chapter would uncover the tactics of combining mountain biking's unique challenges with meditative mindfulness practice, capturing the essence of true serenity in exhilarating motion.

4.1. Experiencing Mindful Cycling

Start by channeling your focus on the current sensations - the winding trail ahead, the texture of the gravel beneath the wheels of your bike, the cool gusts of wind brushing against your skin. Mindfulness requires a complete immersion in the present moment, completely disconnected from the external world's clamor. Make a conscious effort to listen to your bike's rhythmic hum, the crunch of tires rolling over rocks, and leaves rustling in the breeze.

Every successful ride demands an interconnected balance of control - over your gear shifts, your body's synchronization with the bike, understanding the trail's contours, and your mind's unison with your heart's steady rhythm. It's in this control that mindfulness finds its place in mountain biking.

4.2. Unearthing the Edge of Your Focus

Discover the pleasure of concentrating on every turn, every upward climb, and exhilarating downhill dash; the exertion draws you further from the noise of your thoughts, placing you in a state of mindful existence. This pivotal practice doesn't just heighten the richness of your ride; it builds your agility, reaction times, and fosters a deeper grasp of your ongoing experience.

Embrace steady breathing as a means to create a unique rhythm, setting the tempo to adventurous orchestration of bike, body, and terrain. It's a symphony of heartbeats, breaths, and gear shifting that crafts a perfect harmony, fostering an unparalleled sense of tranquility amidst the thrilling activity.

4.3. Conquering the Mountains Mindfully

Climbing steep inclines provides an opportunity to engage in active mindfulness. Muscles straining, slow and focused breathing, the continuous dance of switching gears to maintain momentum, and balancing your body's center of gravity all become elements of a moving meditation. It's extreme physical exertion, yet at the same moment yields an incredible sense of quiet within the mind.

Descending on the other side brings forth exhilaration, a rush waiting to explode from within. Instead of simply succumbing to instinct, try heightening your awareness – sense the changes in landscape, feel the rush of wind, notice the subtle shifts in body weight, and modulate the bike's speed with a unique synchronicity borne from awareness.

Every rise and fall of the trail becomes a mindful challenge to revel in, rather than simply a physical hurdle to surpass.

4.4. Riding Through Transitions

These moments of powerful action transition into pauses – moments of stillness where your heart rate slows, and your breath becomes more regular. Discover the profound beauty in these transitions. They present an opportunity for the mind to revel in tranquility – to detach, reassess, and gently ease back into the rhythm of riding.

These transitions, in essence, serve as checkpoints, alerting you to return your attention inward, refocus and to consciously immerse yourself back into the physical dynamism, hence ensuring the continuity of your mindful ride.

4.5. Nurturing Resilience Along the Trails

Mountain biking tests your limits – the weariness in the legs, the burn in the lungs, and the tension in the muscles. Embrace these challenges with open mindfulness. Use each hurdle as an opportunity to cultivate resilience and develop a deeper understanding of your body's capabilities.

The trail's unpredictability fosters a resilient mindset capable of confronting unexpected problems – a helpful trait both on and off the bike. Sense your constantly evolving growth while embarked on this mindful biking journey.

4.6. Conclusion: An Unending Journey

Every mountain bike ride encapsulates a myriad of emotions and experiences – ones of thrill, of exertion, and profound serenity. Recognize this symbiosis between physical activity and mindful consciousness and construct your own unique biking meditation practice.

The charm lies in the unending journey to self-discovery and improvement – through winding paths, uphill battles, and serene valleys, entirely guided by the balance of motion and mindfulness. Let every ride be a step closer to achieving tranquility, discarding the chaos of the exterior world to uncover an inner cosmos brimming with peace, resilience, and profound understanding.

Chapter 5. Making Meditation Mobile: The Bi-cycle of Awareness

In the pulsating urban jungle, there exists a tranquil haven for zen seekers and fitness freaks alike, stitched together by the pedal strokes of mindful cycling. Welcome to the world of moving meditation, where the bike serves as your mindfulness apparatus, taking you on a ride towards inner peace.

5.1. Merging Meditation and Cycling

Imagine a meditation practice that does not require a quiet room or a comfortable cushion. Instead, you find tranquility while moving at a pace set by your own body and breath, absorbed in the momentum of cycling.

Start by acknowledging that bikes are not merely objects of transport; they are catalysts stirring conversations between your mind, body, and the environment. Respect your bicycle for the flawless weapon of consistency it is, harmonize with its rhythm and let it guide your inner dialogue – the first step to making meditation mobile.

Center yourself in the present moment every time you start to ride. Feel the contact points between you and the bike – your hands on the handlebars, feet on the pedals, and your seating area. Tune in to these sensations and let them anchor you in the experience of riding. The cool rush of air on your face, the rhythmic turning of the wheels, the sounds of the world around you – all serve as stimuli for mindfulness.

5.2. Breathing Patterns and Pedal Cadence

Aligning your breath with the pedal strokes further deepens your connection with cycling. Begin by simply observing your regular breathing pattern and the natural rhythm of your pedaling. After a while, you can start synchronizing them.

A basic practice involves inhaling for two pedal strokes and exhaling for two. As you continue this practice, your breath and cadence become a cyclical meditation mantra that further tunes you into the mindfulness mode. This synchronization also fosters a rhythmic connection between body and mind, reinforcing your awareness of each moment. Incidentally, this alignment aids in improving cycling efficiency – a useful side effect.

Keep in mind that this practice is not about pushing harder or going faster. The focus is on the rhythm, the harmony, and the unity in the whole act of cycling.

5.3. Observation and Non-Judgment

One of the underlying principles of mindfulness is non-judgmental observation. Your cycling route provides plenty of opportunities presented by nature and the urban landscapes. Enjoy those moments, consider them fleeting works of art, and let them flow freely.

As you gaze upon the changing surroundings, refrain from judging what crosses your path. Like clouds drifting across the sky, some visuals might be intriguing, and some might strain your senses. Nonetheless, observe them as they are, let them pass, and concentrate on the road ahead. Absorb the impermanence of these sights, smells, and sounds, enhancing your awareness of the present moment.

5.4. The Uphills and the Downhills of Life

Every ride has its uphills and downhills – much like the journey of life. Seeing them as metaphors, they provide powerful insights to help you cultivate equanimity.

When you are climbing uphill, the instinct is to resist the discomfort. However, consider it an opportunity to practice acceptance and patience. When going downhill, keeping speed in check and navigating wisely requires presence and precision.

In both scenarios, recognize how each pedal stroke, each moment, contributes to the outcome. It's a lesson in cause and effect, an awareness of the continuous flow of life, a reminder that each action resonates well beyond the moment it occurs. Thus, cycling transforms into a mirror reflecting the cycle of life, where awareness of each rise and fall invites enlightened understanding.

5.5. Body Talks: Learning To Listen

Lastly, but most importantly, the body talks during cycling, and it's crucial to listen. It tells you when to slow down and when to energize, when to hydrate, and when to rest. Learning to listen to these subtle cues nurtures a strong connection with your body, thereby fostering holistic wellness.

On this bicycled journey to awareness, pay heed to your body signals – they are your reliable guides to understanding your limits and potentials, an expressive dialogue of self-awareness.

In conclusion, merging mindfulness with cycling grants a unique sense of liberation, intimacy with your inner self, and attentiveness to your surroundings. It's an enriching voyage where each turn of the pedal is an affirmation of life, each ride a journey into personal reflections, and each destination, simply another beginning. Don't just cycle, exist with your ride.

Chapter 6. Tools and Techniques: Pedaling Into Presence

Cycling is not merely an activity, but a place of presence that offers the rhythmic infusion of consciousness with each pedal stroke. Through this section, we will explore various tools and techniques that help you pedal into the realm of mindfulness, transforming each ride into a tranquil journey.

6.1. Observing Your Breathing

Your breathing is the simplest and yet the most profound tool that you can utilize to attain mindfulness while cycling. Observing your breath helps you tune into the present moment and anchor your awareness. It forms the heart of many meditative practices and can be just as effective when adapted for cycling.

While cycling, pay attention to your breath. Notice the inhalation, the momentary pause, and then the exhalation. Observe the rhythm - the pace at which you breathe while you're pushing hard up a hill, or cruising down a slope. Encourage natural and steady breathing, maintaining a balance with your physical exertion.

6.2. Harmonizing Cadence and Breath

Start with this simple practice: try to match your pedal strokes to your breath. Take one complete breath (an inhalation and an exhalation) for a few pedal strokes. This technique encourages conscious effort, rhythm, and tranquility. As you try to match your cycling and breathing rhythms, you will create a moving meditation, a harmony that transcends the mere physical activity.

The longer you maintain this synchronicity, the deeper your connection with the moment becomes, creating an unexpected yet soothing rhythm. Not only does this technique help instill mindfulness, but it also enhances your cycling efficiency and endurance.

6.3. Paying Attention to Your Body

Your focus does not need to be tied exclusively to your breath; mindfulness allows you to expand this awareness to your entire body. As you cycle, become increasingly aware of your body movements. Pay attention to how your feet push down on the pedals, the way your knees bend and extend, or how your hands grip the handlebars.

Notice the sensations in your muscles, how they contract and release, creating the power that propels your bike forward. Feel the wind against your skin, the sun on your back, and the road under your wheels. Not only will this make you more present, but it also helps you respond better to your body's needs, helping prevent strain and injuries.

6.4. Cycling through the Senses

Another technique to bring mindfulness into your ride is to use your five senses. Cycling offers a unique opportunity to engage with the world around you in ways you may not in a more static form of meditation.

Hear: Begin with the auditory sense. Pay attention to sounds — the calming trickles of a passing stream, birdsong, the crunch of gravel under your tires, even the sound of your rhythmic breathing.

See: Look at the visual details around you, the ever-changing scenery as you cycle across various paths and terrains. The dance of shadows and light, color palettes that change with the seasons, or the architectural beauty of the towns you cycle through can all offer moments of presence.

Smell: The olfactory sense can foster an immediate connection with the environment. Whether it's the fresh scent of dewy grass, the mustiness of fallen leaves, the floral aroma of passing flora, or even the earthy scent of a rainy day – each inhale can be a moment of mindfulness.

Taste: This might seem strange initially, but as you get more accustomed to outdoor cycling, you'll start to savor the subtle 'taste' of the environment. This could include the saltiness of sea air if you're cycling along a coastal path, or perhaps, the clean freshness after a sudden rain shower.

Touch: Last but not least, bring awareness to the sensations that your skin picks up. The breathe of wind on your face, the warmth of the sun, the textural differences in your handlebars, the humidity in the air, or the coolness of a passing cloud's shadow — it all extracts you from your busy mind and grounds you to your surroundings.

These techniques ensure that the act of cycling becomes a moving, flowing tapestry of mindfulness, each breath and pedal stroke weaving another thread into your living presence. It's about acknowledging the tension and release within your muscles, the rhythmic dance of your breath, the symphony of senses, and the cycle of exertion and recovery, bringing about a sea change in the way you perceive your rides. Subsequently, this embeds an enhanced sense of tranquility and joy into your two-wheeled travels, helping you maintain a consistent state of serenity amidst the whirl of thoughts.

Stay present, keep pedaling, and find your tranquility on the trail!

Chapter 7. The Subtle Art of Mindful Breathing on the Move

Breathing, the most fundamental aspect of living, often goes unnoticed. Mindful breathing on the move, especially while cycling, yields a transformational sense of awareness and wholeness, linking body, mind, and spirit. This chapter explores the subtle yet profound art of mindful breathing during cycling, teaching one how to extract immense peace and satisfaction from this practice while enhancing one's overall cycling performance.

7.1. Fundamentals of Breathing in Cycling

The act of breathing, so integral to life, shifts in its importance when we engage in strenuous activities. Cycling, particularly, requires an efficient regulation of breath. Understanding the biomechanics of breathing becomes the first step in mastering the mindful art of inhalation and exhalation.

Humans predominantly breathe through the diaphragm, a dome-shaped muscle that contracts and relaxes with every breath we take. Beneath this muscle is our largest organ, the lungs, where vital gas exchange takes place. During intense sessions of cycling, the demand for oxygen increases, manifesting in quicker, shorter breaths. However, mindful breathing techniques promote a shift from this shallow chest breathing to deep or diaphragmatic breathing, which enhances the volume of oxygen intake and elicits a sense of calm.

7.2. Introduction to Mindful Breathing

Mindful breathing is an ancient practice that signifies being present in the moment, appreciating each breath we take. It encourages individuals to delve into a profoundly personal space, fostering tranquility and mindfulness. Incorporating mindful breathing into cycling transforms the ride into a holistically beneficial experience. A pattern of controlled, deep breaths, maintained throughout the ride, uplifts the spirit and fortifies the focus, creating a deep bond between the cyclist and their journey.

7.3. Technique of Performing Mindful Breathing

1. Begin with a comfortable and well-aligned cycling position. A relaxed posture not only boosts performance but also facilitates easier breathing, as it prevents constricting the lungs or diaphragm.

2. As you pedal, shift your focus on your breathing pattern. Place a hand on your abdomen to feel the rising and falling motion as you take in a breath and exhale it. This conscious awareness of your breath is the stepping stone towards mindful breathing.

3. Establish a rhythm between your breath and pedaling. A commonly used pattern amongst cyclists is inhaling for two pedal strokes and exhaling for two. This pattern may be adjusted to suit your comfort and requirement, though maintaining a rhythm is crucial.

4. Aim for even, deep breaths into the belly rather than shallow, chest-level breaths. Deep breathing encourages the maximum intake of oxygen, keeps muscles adequately oxygenated, and fosters relaxation during the ride.

7.4. The Art of Synchronized Breathing and Pedalling

There exists a potent connection between our breaths and physical activity. Synchronizing our breaths with the motion of pedaling harnesses this connection, leading to a rhythmic flow that fills our cycling experience with calm energy.

1. Start to establish a breathing rhythm that corresponds to your pedaling cadence. For instance, inhale during upstrokes and exhale during downstrokes. Primarily, the inhalation and exhalation periods should match the effort exerted during the cycle strokes.

2. Maintain the synchronicity. Irregularities in pace can disrupt the breath-pedal rhythm. Practice maintaining a steady speed to uphold the continuity of your breaths, enhancing your overall cycling experience.

3. Concentrate on the breath-pedal sync. Use it as a meditation tool to divert your mind from unwanted distractions. It induces a state of 'flow' where you and the cycle move as a unified entity.

7.5. The Benefits and Impact of Mindful Breathing

Mindful breathing during cycling offers several benefits for the body, mind, and spirit alike.

1. Performance Enhancement: With an abundant oxygen supply to muscles, riders have noticed significant improvements in their cycling stamina and speed.

2. Tranquility and Relaxation: The act of fully engaging with one's breath brings about a calming effect. It lowers stress levels, fights fatigue, and introduces a state of Zen during your cycling

adventure.

3. Enhanced Awareness: Mindful breathing also helps create a heightened sense of self and surrounding awareness. As we focus on our breath, we tune out other distractions, amplifying our perception of the self and our connection with the surrounding environment.

In conclusion, integrating mindful breathing into your cycling routine holds the potential to transform the mere act of riding a bicycle into a pathway to inner peace and heightened performance. As you master this art, you may identify the rhythm that exists everywhere - in nature, inside you, in the universe. This rhythm, powered by your breath, can make your journey not just about the destination, but about every pedal stroke and every breath. It's not just cycling, it's a mode of discovery, exploration, and profound joy.

Chapter 8. Harnessing Nature's Bounty: The Mental Landscapes of Cycling

The romance between a cyclist and the road often seems like a quiet conversation with nature. Like an internal pilgrimage, the endless expanse in front of us invites self-reflection, granting passage through the winding roads of our minds as much as the terrain. This chapter invites you to delve into the concept of cycling not just as a physical activity, but as a deeply spiritual journey that is empowered by nature and its bounties.

8.1. The Rhythmic Poetry of the Pedal

With each pedal stroke, there is an unspoken rhythm. Hear the symphony that the cranks, chain, and wheels form, accompanied by the gentle whisper of the wind and the subtle crunch of the gravel. Feel the cadence - free and unburdened, like the heartbeat of the road itself. This is where mindfulness begins, turning an act of muscle and sweat into a dance of serenity.

Each ride, especially when taken with the purpose of mindfulness, morphs into a meditative session. The road becomes your muse and your mind the poet, cycling itself turns into rhythmic poetry, where every spin of the wheel is a verse written in the stretch of tarmac or the mountain trail.

8.2. Embracing the Blur of Scenery

As you cycle, the scenery around you blends into a multiple exposure snapshot, a humbling reminder of life's transitory nature and the passage of time. One moment it's the sprawling cityscape, the next a serene lake or the unflinching mountains. Anchoring your attention to this constant change keeps your mind centered in the present moment.

In the seeming blur of changing landscapes, let each breath sync with the revolution of your wheels, grounding you in the here and now. It's not just about the destination but the journey and the many landscapes it traverses - both, external and internal.

8.3. The Metaphorical Journey

Cycling is more than the literal journey from one point to another. It also maps a metaphorical journey within ourselves. Each ride is a fresh expedition into our inner world, every hill climbed a victory over a personal fear, every mile covered an affirmation of our resilience.

The road's ascents, descents, bends, and straights are gentle reminders of life's ebb and flow, the challenges and victories, the changes and consistencies. Just as you navigate your bike through these physical landscapes, so too are you navigating through the mental landscapes of your life.

8.4. The Restorative Power of Nature

Cycling immerses you in the nurturing embrace of nature. The feeling of the wind against your face, the range of colors as the sun sets or rises, the smells of wet earth or blooming flowers, all contribute to the creation of a multisensory palette that rejuvenates mind and body alike.

Inhaling fresh air, engaging with the changing terrain, and absorbing the surrounding beauty activates the senses in a way that no indoor activity can. The act of cycling thus yields a unique form of therapy, an active meditation that harnesses the restorative power of nature.

8.5. Conclusion: The Congruence of Body, Mind, and Nature

Every time you straddle the saddle, remember that a ride is more than the physical distance covered or calories burnt. The bike is a vessel, not just transporting you across physical space, but into the depths of your mind, charting new territories of self-awareness, joy, and tranquility.

Taking the time to savor and engage with these physical and mental landscapes can transform your ride into a spiritual journey, where each pedal stroke builds a bridge between your inner and outer worlds. By harnessing nature's bounty and the mental landscapes of cycling, you can achieve a harmonious state of mindfulness, anchoring within you an enduring sense of serenity.

Remember, in the grand scheme of things, we all are cyclists in our own right - cycling through life, learning, growing, pushing through, and evolving with every revolution. The next time you hop onto your bike, try not just to cycle, but to dance with the flow of life and experience the true essence of 'Cycled Serenity'.

Chapter 9. From Adrenaline to Zen: Reshaping The Rider's Experience

We begin this exploration teetering on the edge of excitement, anxious anticipation bubbling within us as we prepare for our ascent — both literal and metaphysical. The act of mounting the bike, pressing foot to pedal, and pushing forward is more than the start of a journey. It's the commencement of a profound transformation that blends the physical and spiritual, effortlessly marrying the thrill of cycling with the peace of mindfulness. We're transcending the realms of typical cycling guides, veering off the beaten path to unite the world of meditation and mindfulness with the realm of road cycling and mountain biking.

==="" Physical Preparation: Launching the Journey "

First, it is vital to consider physical readiness. Just as you wouldn't run a marathon without training, you shouldn't undertake mindful cycling without preparing your body. A solid base of physical fitness serves as a springboard to your spiritual journey, allowing you to focus less on the strain of the activity and more on the metaphysical aspect.

A regular cycling routine that consists of varying intensities and terrains can be a good starting point. Utilize strength training and stretching exercises to complement this, focusing on areas primarily used during cycling –legs and core. These activities prevent injury, increase endurance, and promote better control over your bike, prerequisites for smoothly transitioning into mindful cycling.

==="" Mindful Preparation: Setting Inward Intentions "

Arguably more critical than your physical preparedness is your mental readiness. Before initiating your ride, engage in a few moments of focused meditation to clear your mind of distractions and set your intentions for the ride.

This meditation doesn't need to be complicated. Closing your eyes, deep breaths, and focusing your mind on the cycling journey ahead is enough. Visualize yourself cycling, the rhythm of your pedals, the wind against your skin, the scenic panorama unfolding as you progress. This exercise lessens the initial resistance, grounding you into the moment, and aligns your focus towards your impending transformation.

==="The Ascent: Transcending Physical Limits"

Ascending on your bicycle offers valuable lessons in endurance, determination, and resilience. The upward climb, while physically challenging, is symbolic; it represents your spiritual rise, your ascension beyond everyday stress and chaos, into a state of serenity and clarity.

When you feel the burn in your muscles and the strain on your breath, don't retract in discomfort. Lean into it, become aware of these sensations. Welcome this adversity as an integral part of your journey. This mindfulness will help you embrace and appreciate the effort you're exerting, turning a potentially negative experience into an enlightening one.

==="Descend with Awareness: Finding Serenity in Release"

Then comes the much-anticipated descent, the thrilling reward for your arduous uphill trek. Yet, the real reward is the opportunity to realize mindfulness during the exhilarating speed and rush of adrenaline. As your bike effortlessly glides downwards, allow your awareness to anchor onto your body and the sensations around you.

Feel the pressure lessening on your thighs, the swift, cooling wind improving your breath, the excited whoosh of your heartbeat, and the thrill that sparks within your veins. Engage all senses, from the rumbling beneath your tires to the panoramic view that rushes past. Maintaining this strong sense of awareness, even amidst the whirlwind of sensations, helps you tap into a profound calmness beneath the exhilaration.

===" Completing the Cycle: Integrating Physical Exertion and Mindful Tranquility "

As your cycling route ebbs and flows, with ascents and descents offering their unique challenges and rewards, begin to recognize the rhythm of your journey. This rhythm isn't just the physical act of pedaling—it's the pulsating heart of your mindful cycling experience, the interconnected cycle of exertion and tranquility, effort and release, adrenaline and zen.

Understand, now, how this cycle mirrors life and its oscillating nature: the constant interplay of hard work and reward, struggle and victory, chaos and serenity.

Explore this concept further by integrating it into your rides. Start by noticing your breath and how it fluctuates between vigorous climbs and effortless descents. Later, focus on syncing your breath with your pedaling rhythm, creating a harmonious synthesis of breath, body, and bike, an embodiment of the physical and mental balance you seek.

===" Post-Ride Reflection: Translating Insight into Action "

Once the rhythmic pedaling slows and the ride concludes, your experience doesn't end. Instead, you're presented with a priceless opportunity: to reflect on your journey and extract insights that can be applied to everyday life.

Ask yourself: What was different with mindful cycling? Did you perceive your physical exertion differently? Were you more aware of your thoughts and feelings? Did the overall experience change?

These questions anchor the insights gained during your ride to your overall mindfulness practice.

When you begin to realize that mindfulness principles can be applied as effectively on a bustling street as a mountain trail, you arrive at the crux of zen. Having linked the chaotic elements of the physical world (cycling) to the calm, internal world (mindfulness), you've transcended the barriers of traditional cycling, reshaping your cycling and life experience from a pursuit of adrenaline to an ascension towards serenity. This, dear rider, marks your true metamorphosis from a cyclist to a mindful rider, opening a new chapter in your journey towards holistic well-being.

Chapter 10. Roadblocks and resilience: Overcoming Mental Hurdles on the Trail

Building resilience is an essential part of every cyclist's journey. The road ahead can often unconsciously divert our focus from the adventure at hand, to fear and anxiety. Such mental hurdles could hinder our progress, and sometimes, even discourage us completely. Overcoming these mental roadblocks fosters resilience, an integral attribute that empowers us not just to ride better, but to live better. This chapter sheds light on recognizing and overcoming these mental hurdles, paving the way for a more resilient excursion.

10.1. Identifying Mental Roadblocks

Mental roadblocks come in as many forms as the trails we tread. Anxiety about the road ahead, self-doubt about personal physical abilities, and an obsession with results often cloud the joyful experience of cycling. Moreover, extrinsic factors such as peer pressure, performance comparisons, and extreme weather conditions add to the mix, making it even more crucial to identify these mental roadblocks early on.

One way to recognize these hurdles is by maintaining a 'Ride Journal.' This journal not only helps you track your progress but also helps identify patterns. Reflecting on your journal entries can reveal recurring obstacles or roadblocks that hamper the cycling experience, effectively helping you address them.

10.2. Taming Anxiety

Anxiety ahead of a ride can sap our energy even before we embark on the trail. Leading psychologists opine that shifting the focus from the fear of a potential outcome to the process can significantly reduce pre-ride anxiety. This means relishing the sensation of wind against your face, observing the rhythmic pattern of your breath, and experiencing the movements of your body during the ride as opposed to primarily focusing on performance.

Relaxation techniques such as deep breathing or practicing a short cycle of mindfulness meditation before the ride can also prove beneficial in managing anxiety. Visualize yourself navigating the course with ease and confidence.

10.3. Combatting Self-Doubt

Doubting one's abilities does not yield progress; rather, it clangs the chains that bind us to stagnation. It is alright to fail and falter sometimes. Use these moments to discern areas of improvement rather than seeing them as indicators of your capabilities. You could perhaps work on enhancing your endurance or mastering the art of braking smoothly.

Remember, every champion cyclist started as a novice. They fell, grazed their knees, dusted off, and persisted. Acknowledge your progress, however small, and shower yourself with the deserving praise. A pat on the back goes a long way in bolstering self-confidence.

10.4. Dealing with Obsession over Results

Sometimes we get so blinded by results that we forget to enjoy the ride. This relentless pursuit of outcomes robs us of the joy inherent in cycling. Cycling mindfully puts you back in sync with the immediate experience and helps disentangle from the obsessive pursuit of results. Stay attentive to enjoy the rhythmic harmony of pedaling, inhale the stinging cold air, and relish the unfolding scenic beauty. Remember, the journey is as essential as the destination.

10.5. Overcoming Extrinsic Pressure

Peer pressure and performance comparisons can add an unnecessary burden, affecting your performance negatively. Understand that every cyclist has a unique journey characterized by unique strengths and areas of improvement. Redirect your focus from competition to personal improvement. Seek support from your cycling community but remember that your ride, your pace, and your progress belong only to you.

10.6. Bracing Against Harsh Conditions

Harsh weather conditions may demotivate even the most ardent cyclists. However, using the right gear can boost your comfort and performance under such conditions. Invest in warm and waterproof clothing for cold, wet days and lighter, breathable wear for hotter condition. Remember, there's no such thing as bad weather, just inappropriate clothing.

In conclusion, overcoming mental roadblocks is about embracing every stumble, learning from it, and riding ahead with unwavering determination. It's about finding joy in the grueling ascents and not just the freewheeling descents. It's about resilience, an unflappable resolve that propels you further than you ever thought possible with each pedal stroke. The trails will always change, the weather will always surprise, and the obsessions and doubts may linger, but armed with resilience, every ride becomes a harmonious symphony of mental strength and physical prowess.

Chapter 11. Cycling Tales: Inspirational Stories of Mindful Cyclists

As our wheels touch the tarmac, or hum along the ruffled dirt of a well-trodden mountain trail, so they spin stories. These are the narratives of the cyclists who have embraced the path of mindfulness. Their tales seep into the grooves of their tire treads, written with every mindful pedal stroke, and they are here to inspire you.

11.1. Unleashing Inner Stillness amidst Motion: John's Journey

John used to be an anxious employee, always running the rat race. One day, while stuck in bumper-to-bumper traffic, he chanced upon a cyclist, breezing past the line of cars. Instead of envy, he felt admiration—the cyclist's effortless glides were like poetry in motion.

Thus began John's journey into cycling. Every morning, he headed out for a ride. Soon, he realized that the road was not just a path but a conduit for his thoughts. The rhythmic pedaling became a calming mantra, quieting his racing mind. And with each breath, he unlocked a new level of tranquility, cycling not away from, but into an oasis of inner peace amidst the bustling city.

John was no longer just a participant in the rat race; he cycled above it, on a higher plane of mindful consciousness.

11.2. Embracing the Ebb and Flow: Cathy's Conquest

Cathy was passionate about mountain biking. She found beauty in her struggle against the rugged, twisting trails of nature. However, mountain biking left its toll on her body and mind. The constant focus on overcoming obstacles created a perpetual tension, both mentally and physically.

Through mindfulness, she discovered a new way to approach trail rides. She allowed the ebb and flow of the mountain to guide her. Cathy learned to absorb the impact of each rock or root, using the momentum to power her forward, instead of resisting it.

It became a dance of sorts—every bump, every curve were dance steps, every struggle was a rhythm, and she flowed with it. The trail was no longer a battlefield, but a dance floor. The mindful cycling technique taught Cathy to embrace the ebb and flow of life itself, and she felt more at peace than ever before.

11.3. Road to Recovery: Elizabeth's Evolution

After a car accident, Elizabeth found herself grappling with chronic pain. Cycling became her refuge. Initially, every pedal stroke was a painful reminder of her accident.

However, as she started using mindful techniques, the pains of the episode started receding. Elizabeth began to focus on her breathing, on the feeling of the wind brushing her skin, and the sound of her chain gently humming along with her pace. Each moment became an opportunity to let go of the suffering and embrace joy.

It was on one of these rides that the breakthrough happened. The pain was there, but it no longer held power over her. By acknowledging the presence of pain rather than resisting it, Elizabeth learned through mindful cycling to regain control over her life. She was no longer a victim of circumstances but a resilient survivor. Cycling served as her road to recovery—a journey towards healing.

John, Cathy, and Elizabeth's stories are but a few examples of the transformative journey that mindful cycling brings about—a change not just within the riders but radiating outwards affecting their everyday life. Mindful cycling allows the rider to appreciate life's simple yet profound moments, invoking serenity within. By harnessing the power of cycling, these pedal-powered philosophers invite you to experience tranquility on two wheels.

Cycling offers us a unique space to connect with ourselves and the world around us. With mind, body, and soul in harmony, the simple act of pedaling becomes something far more significant—a mindful practice, a meditation, an exploration into the depth of our own consciousness.

Whether you're traversing majestic mountains or conquering urban jungles, every journey can be an enlightened voyage into your soul's tranquility. The key is to cycle with mindfulness. So gear up, and let's cycle into serenity.